MENSTRUAL
DOODLES

Dedicated to my clever, wonderful daughter Clara, who taught me how important it is to enjoy being a woman.

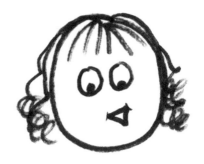

MENSTRUAL DOODLES

DR BECKY MARTIN

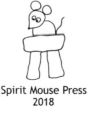

Spirit Mouse Press
2018

First Printing: 2018

ISBN 9-780244-712853

Spirit Mouse Press, UK
spiritmousepress.com

Contents

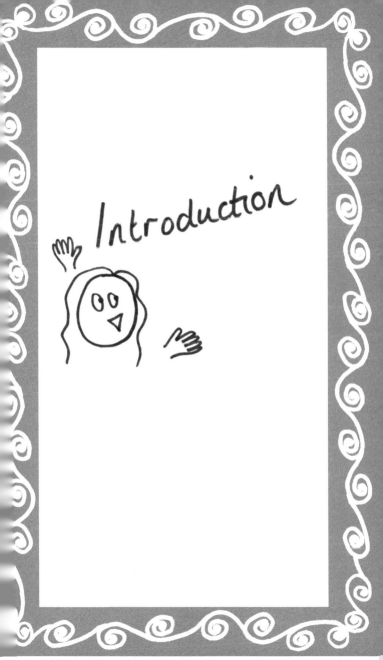

Introduction

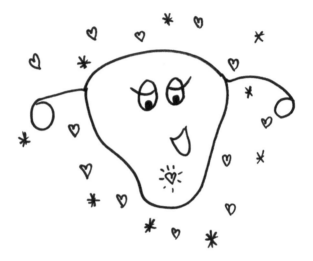

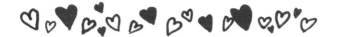

I want to share a secret with you - a secret I did not learn until I was in my mid-thirties. The secret is... drum roll, please... the menstrual cycle is an amazing gift that goes way beyond child-bearing potential. Periods can be pleasurable and every month your body can teach you new things about life, love and the universe.

Crazy, right? But it's true!

This book is an expression of my joy at all I have learnt about my womb and her wonderful workings. Some doodles may resonate with you and some may not; it's important to remember we all have different experiences of life, but I hope there is something for everyone within these pages.

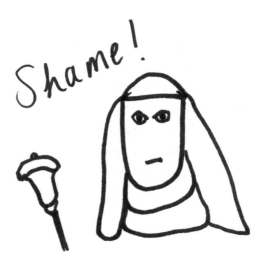

Shame!

Women have been shamed for menstruating for millennia. We are starting to heal now but those wounds run deep. It's still a taboo subject. History was written by the victors, but we are finally getting a chance to write HerStory now. Enough is enough. Let's break the taboo and celebrate the power of the womb.

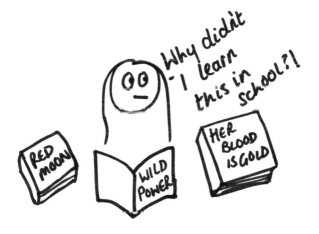

Most people get the dry biology talk in school, but very little practical help on how to utilise their menstrual cycle for better living, or how to spot when things are going astray.

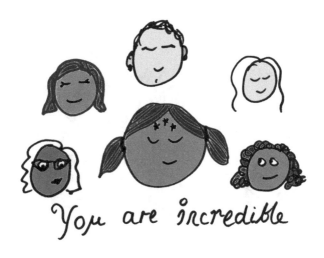

You are incredible

You are incredible. Don't ever forget that. There are women all around you who care about you; mothers, sisters, teachers, aunties, friends. If you have any problems with your periods, reach out, and don't stop searching until you find the peace and dignity you deserve. Together we can smash the taboos and make menstruation a happy place.

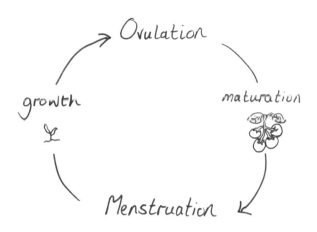

Ovulation

growth

maturation

Menstruation

The two main events in the menstrual cycle are ovulation, when an ovum is released, and menstruation (period), when womb lining is shed. In the follicular phase (menstruation to ovulation) womb lining cells multiply. In the luteal phase (post-ovulation to menstruation) the lining matures, becoming ready to accept a fertilised egg.

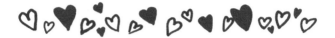

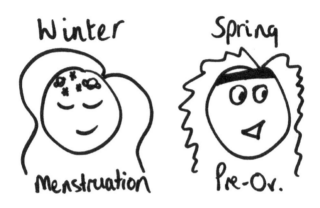

Winter — Menstruation

Spring — Pre-Ov.

Introducing the inner seasons of the menstrual cycle. We shed our womb lining during menstruation, the dying-off of winter. New growth starts again in spring until our eggs are ready to be fertilised in the summer of ovulation.

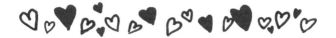

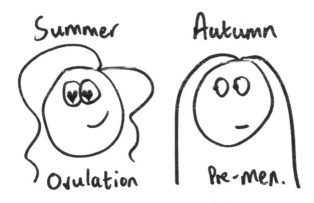

Summer — Ovulation

Autumn — Pre-men.

Womb lining ripens throughout autumn, the post-ovulation/premenstrual phase (luteal phase). The winter of menstruation then comes around again, or successful pregnancy is achieved. We experience four seasons in one month.

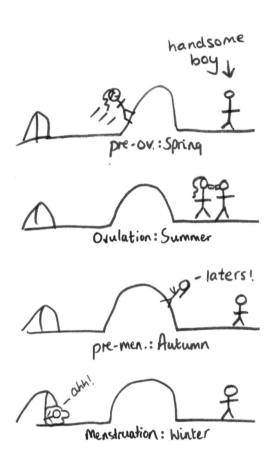

What causes the inner seasons to come about? Hormones, mostly.

Our bodies are incredible. They perform such an intricate dance, affecting energy levels, mood and behaviours to bring about successful fertilisation.

We are not slaves to our biology; we can ignore it and crack on, but why swim against the stream if you don't have to?

Menstrual cycle tracking is so much fun!

Note each day how you are feeling in body, mind and spirit.

Observe the changing of the seasons. See difficult days coming instead of being surprised by them. Look forward to the fun bits and predict when the bad bits will pass. Be ready to face the challenges, and each cycle learn more about yourself and your world.

The ultimate mindfulness practise for those of us lucky enough to have wombs.

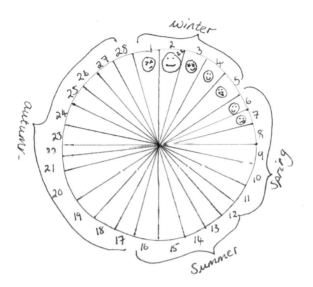

How are you feeling today?

- grumpy
- sad
- happy
- energetic
- tired
- creative
- sexual

- analytical
- focused
- dreamy
- meditative
- sensual
- productive
- reflective

We are all a bit different!

Day 1

Day 8

Day 14

Day 21

We are all a bit different. We all experience the menstrual cycle in our own way. This book covers the more common experiences, but it varies widely between people and between cycles. The only way to see what's going on with you is to track feelings, moods and sensations daily.

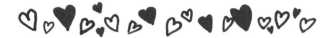

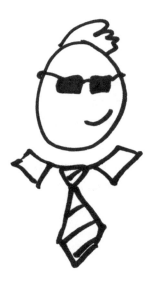

Some people who menstruate do not identify as women. Everyone with a womb deserves love, help with menstrual issues and fabulous menstrual products.

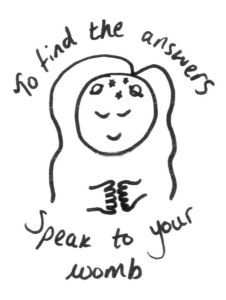

To find the answers Speak to your womb

This might sound bonkers at first, but stick with it. Put your hands on your lower belly, close your eyes and bring your focus to your womb. Say hello. Ask her how she is. Be still and wait for a response. Observe any images that come to mind, any feelings that arise. Be open to whatever she has to say.

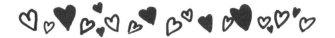

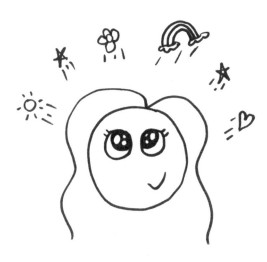

I hope that by the time you finish this book, you will feel great about your menstrual cycle. By working with your cycle I hope you will find more ways to be kind to yourself and to live a fuller, more creative life so that when you think of your womb you will feel the pure, blissful happiness that you deserve.

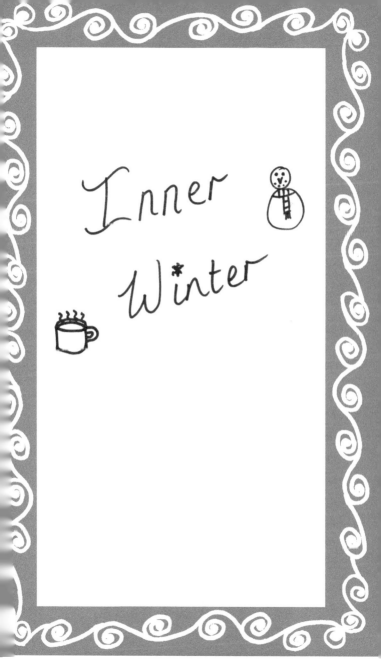

Inner Winter

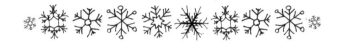

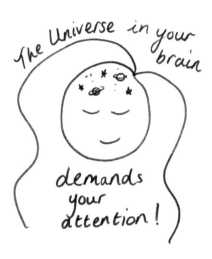

Menstruation is a time to rest and connect with your inner world. Most people do not feel energetic during their bleed and common symptoms such as pain and irritability could be a call to rest and retreat. A day or two of minimal activity at the beginning of your period can profoundly increase productivity during the rest of the cycle.

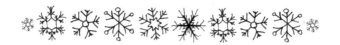

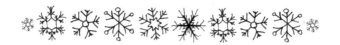

I've got your back

pre-men.: Autumn

uhh!

Menstruation: Winter

he's a keeper!

Partners who support our need to retreat during menstruation are the best.

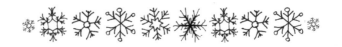

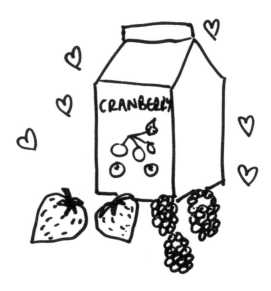

Honouring your bleed can revolutionise your life and turn a painful inconvenience into an empowered pleasure. Possible ways to do this: meditation, making music, eating red food, minimal device time, long baths and saying no to anything that requires physical or emotional energy. Find what works for you.

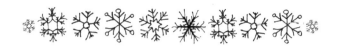

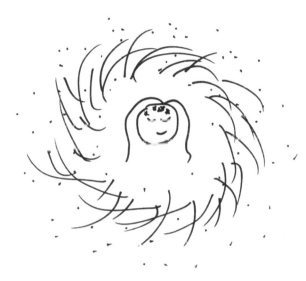

I love the ease with which I can slip into a meditative trance during menstruation. That blissful state of consciousness is there, ready and waiting. Failing to heed the call can cause irritability. It's our birthright as women. It's our gift. It's powerful and game changing. All the wisdom and answers lie there. Reclaim it. Menstruation is not a curse; it is a marvellous gift.

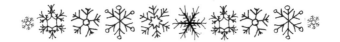

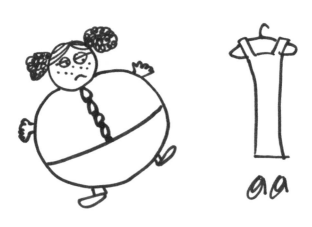

Sometimes we can feel quite bloated during our bleed. Putting on glad rags and going out can seem like a chore.

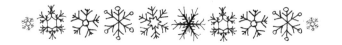

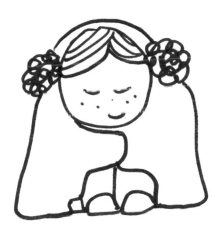

Why not cuddle up in your favourite blanket and chill instead?

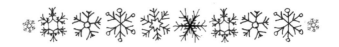

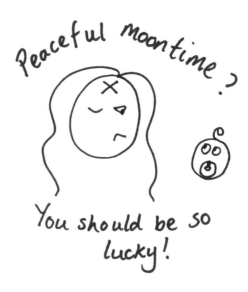

Peaceful moontime?

You should be so lucky!

Looking after kids whilst trying to have a peaceful, meditative bleed is nigh on impossible. Applying cartoons liberally could make for better parenting the rest of the month.

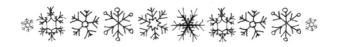

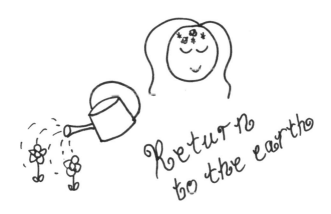

Return to the earth

Menstrual fluid is an excellent fertiliser for plants.
Returning our blood to the earth helps remind us
we are a part of nature and not separate from it.
A simple, discreet method is to rinse cloth pads in
a bowl of water then transfer to a watering can.

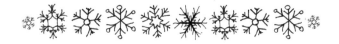

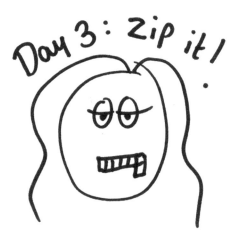

A burst of unexpected energy can come towards the end of your bleed, and the impulse to act or speak up can be strong. Like the first shoots of early spring, you may encounter a later frost, and find yourself feeling raw and vulnerable after creative conflicts. Holding back for a few days longer can help.

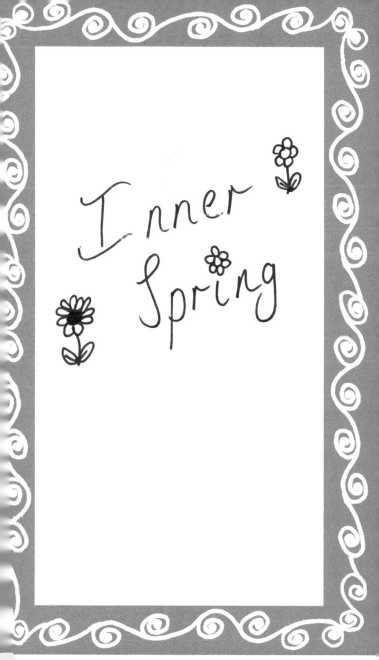

Inner
Spring

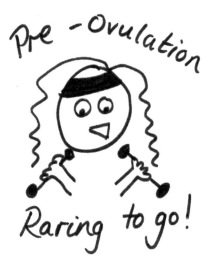

Pre - Ovulation

Raring to go!

As oestrogen levels start to rise after menstruation in inner spring, energy levels rise. This time of renewed vigour and fresh outlook can be great for starting new projects or ventures.

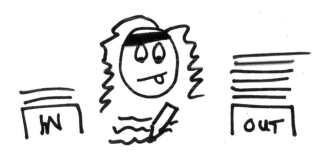

Every cycle in inner spring I have a day when I am mega focused. I can get so much done but it has to be a task that demands single-mindedness. For some reason it is easier to find space for this energy than carving time out for rest.

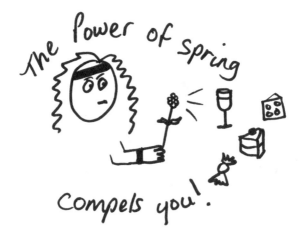

The Power of spring compels you!

Kicking addictions such as sugar and alcohol can be challenging. Inner spring is a great time to start. Energy levels and determination are high and the more experience you have under your belt before you hit the cravings of inner autumn (premenstrual time), the better.

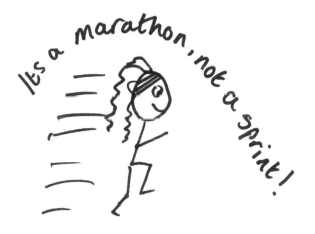

It's a marathon, not a sprint!

After emerging from the cocoon of winter, it can be tempting to burst out of the blocks and race for gold. If you often find yourself exhausted by the end of your cycle, taking it a little bit easier in spring might help. Listening to your body can involve observations over a whole cycle.

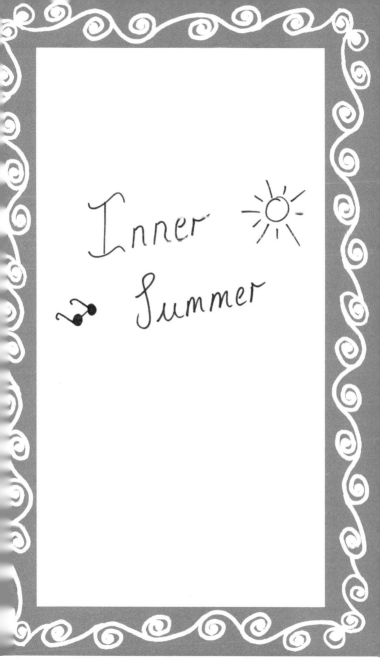

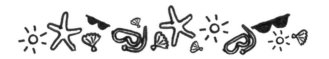

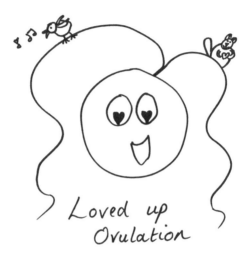

Loved up
Ovulation

Ovulation is great! Oxytocin (the love hormone) levels are high. Our ability to empathise and connect with others is strong. The menstrual cycle is about so much more than periods (although they can be wonderful too!). Ovulation is the high point for many.

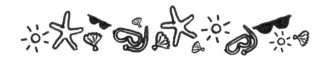

A word of caution: in the gorgeous glow of ovulation it is tempting to say yes to everything and everyone. Take care not to over stretch yourself, as energy levels often fall after ovulation to some degree and you may regret signing up for so much.

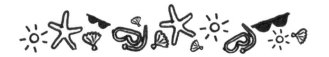

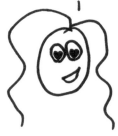

My ex isn't
so bad...

Ovulation

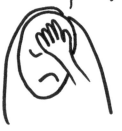

What was I
thinking!

post ovulation

During the ovulatory phase, inner summer, when hormone feel-good levels are high, your body can conspire against you to get pregnant. Be careful of making decisions that your inner autumn wouldn't approve of. She is just around the corner waiting for you with her arms crossed and her army of inner critic demons ready to pounce.

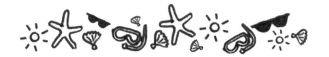

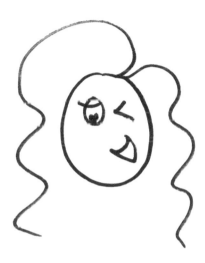

Inner summer, she's a bit of a one. She's high on hormones and says yes a lot. Yes, Yes, Yes! She can get you in trouble but she has her own wisdom, giving you confidence to reach out and make connections that will fulfil you all cycle round. She dares you to live life to the full.

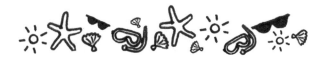

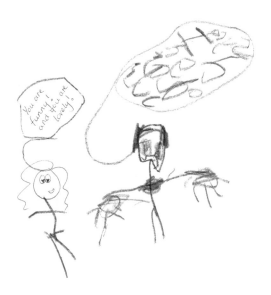

My son thought my doodles were lacking two things, bodies and boys, so he fixed this one for me. The boy is saying, 'I've had enough of having long arms'. Kids are cute in inner summer. He dictated the response. It's the time of the month I find parenting the easiest.

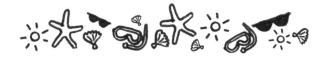

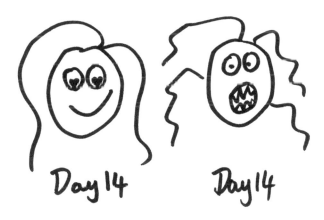

Day 14   Day 14

Another reminder: we are all a bit different. For some women inner summer can be a cranky time. The doodles in this book focus on the more frequent experiences or my personal experiences. It's important to let go of expectations; merely observe and make notes. It's the mindfulness that really matters, being centred within your body and responding to what it needs.

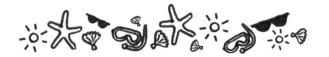

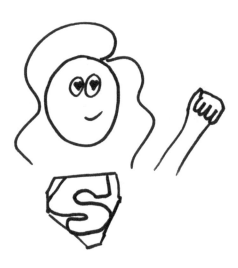

The more I observe my menstrual cycle the more it seems that inner autumn (premenstrual period) is my 'normal' time and the rest of the month I have extra super powers. It's just the coming down from the highs that is hard to hack. At least, if you are menstrual cycle aware, you know you are on the ride, as opposed to just being taken for a ride.

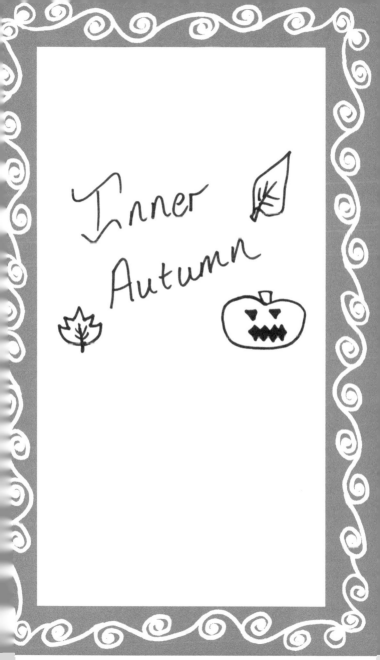

Inner

Autumn

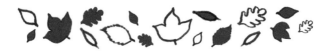

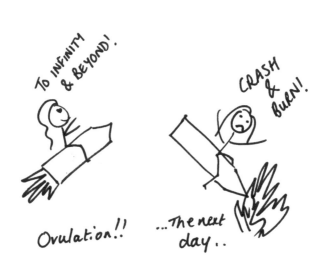

To INFINITY & BEYOND!

CRASH & BURN!

Ovulation!!

...The next day..

A sudden drop in hormone levels can bring the summer party to an abrupt end. The post-ovulation hangover is the worst day of the cycle for some. It's the knee-jerk element that is difficult to cope with; that moment when the trip turns bad. What lessons are there? It's not surprising it can be a rough ride; all of a sudden your body has to heat you up by half a degree!

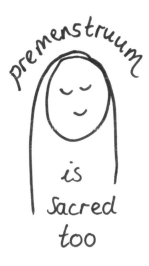

premenstruum is sacred too

At ovulation we release an egg. The next two weeks are a beautiful time in the female body. It's a time of nurturing and protection of the hope of life. If fertilisation has occurred, implantation must follow. Our wombs take a spark and build a fire. We are called to take more care of ourselves, prioritising our own well-being. Holding space for your body to be what it needs to be at this sacred time can bring great peace.

You took my
last biscuit,
oh ok,
nevermind

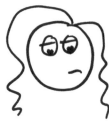

You've been talking
about yourself
for hours,
oh ok,
nevermind

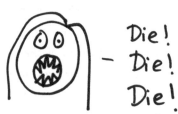

Die!
Die!
Die!

The premenstrual phase calls us to address all the issues we have pushed to one side during the rest of the month. Things we have tolerated up until now become unbearable. Your body is calling you to rearrange your life to be more kind to YOU. She is wise; listen to her. It can be the most challenging season, but it's where so much gold lies.

Premenstruum

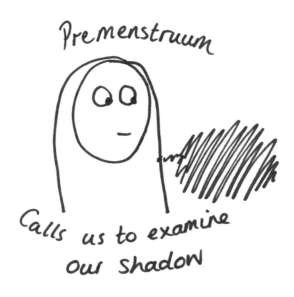

Calls us to examine our shadow

For many, the premenstrual time is a time for reflection. Analytical skills are heightened and focus turns inwards. Whether you like it or not, issues can come to the fore at this time.

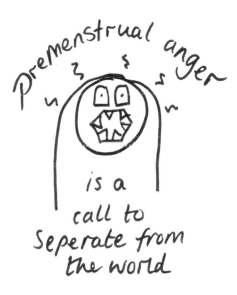

Premenstrual anger is a call to Seperate from the world

In order to do the internal work we are called to do during inner autumn, we may need to isolate ourselves to some degree from our world and the people in it. Premenstrual anger can occur when we do not answer the call for solitude. If mood swings are a problem for you at this time, try carving more 'alone time' out of your schedule.

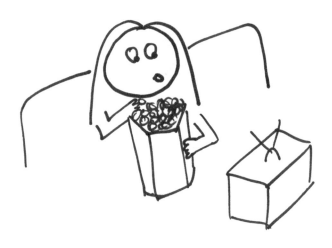

It is common for energy levels to fall somewhat in inner autumn. Everyone is different, but if the only exercise you feel like doing at this time is hand-to-mouth, you wouldn't be alone.

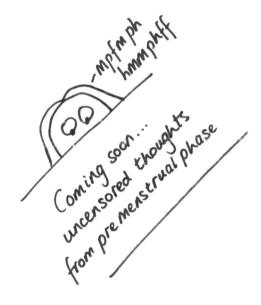

Sometimes I don't trust my premenstrual self's judgement because she can be so negative. I'm taking a note of everything she says and I'm going to bleed on it. When I've finished bleeding, I'll come back to her thoughts and deal with them.

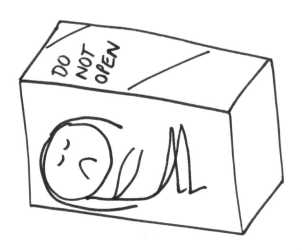

It's easier to love our highly socialised, more pleasant seasons. But the radical honesty and righteous anger of the inner autumn phase play a vital role in making the world a better place. What do we lose when we put her in a box?

She's the game changer of the cycle. She's the one who shakes things up. She's the fire in the belly that drives positive change. We are conditioned to fear her though. She makes you crazy; she's destructive etc.

Can we change our feelings about her emergence? Can we lift the lid so she doesn't have to hurt herself on the way out?

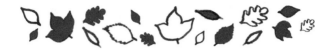

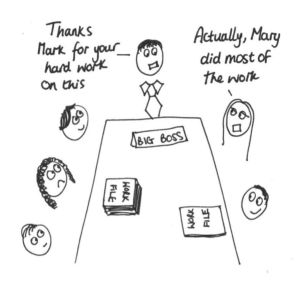

The revolutionary fire in the belly of our inner autumn can take us to scary places. She drives us to make the changes needed to improve our environment in all aspects of life, including the workplace.

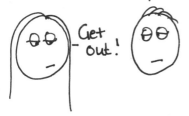

..and home.

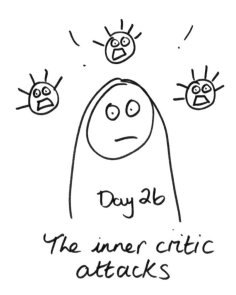

Day 26

The inner critic attacks

Your inner critic can have a field day in the premenstrual part of your cycle.

Befriending the inner critic

Our inner critic can make our lives hellish. But deep down she has our best interests at heart. She wants to protect us from pain and social exclusion. She just doesn't know when to stop. What is she trying to tell you? What can you learn from her? Can you say to her 'thank you for your concern, but don't worry; I am just fine'?

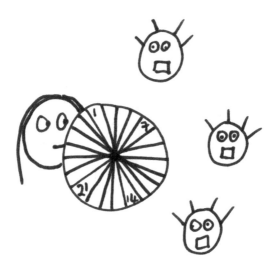

Recording your thoughts and feelings every day is a fabulous practise to get in touch with your menstrual cycle and become more present in your body. You can spot the days when your inner critic is most active and have coping strategies lined up; have lots of nourishing activities planned and be ready to be really kind to yourself.

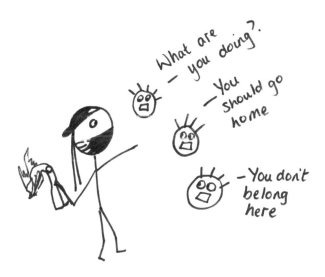

The revolutionary flame and the inner critic are the yin and yang of inner autumn. Learning to balance and utilise them effectively is a life-long challenge. Both have their roots in discernment. Both bring gifts of incredible wisdom once you learn to master their immense presence and potential.

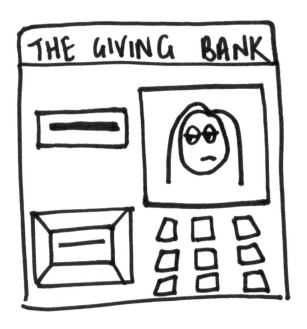

Women are socialised to be givers. We are expected to give our time, energy and emotional labour without consideration for our own needs or wants. In the spring/summer phases this is just about bearable, but in the autumn/winter phases we often need to withdraw and conserve our energy for ourselves.

Unfortunately, society fails to recognise this (or even to acknowledge why expecting so much of women in general is unfair!). It's one of the reasons why menstrual cycle education is so important for the mental health and well-being of women and girls.

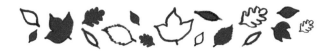

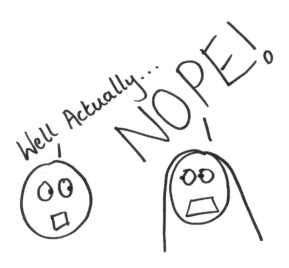

Women are expected to tolerate things men never tolerate. The frustration builds up and won't be kept in the shadows come premenstrual time. Having firm boundaries throughout the month can ease the difficulties of inner autumn to a huge degree.

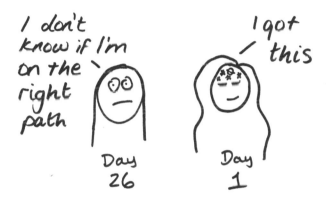

Feeling doubt about the direction of your life is normal in inner autumn. It's part of the analysis and reflection process we go through. With a bit of luck and a lot of support we can get the down-time we need in menstruation. The answers will then flow with the blood. It can feel like a long wait sometimes.

Day 8

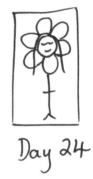

Day 24

The creative process can be strongly influenced by the menstrual cycle. The energy and enthusiasm of spring can bring a burst of new ideas. The reflective depths of autumn can bring you to some very deep places; not just making art, but becoming one with the art. That disclaimer again: everyone is a bit different!

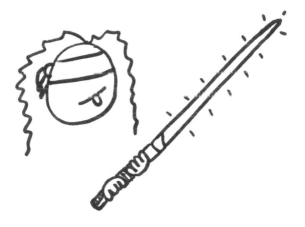

Allow your ideas to experience the full work-up of inner autumn, turning them inside out and upside down. A good bleed with plenty of space and time can allow you to drop into yourself and download updates from the mainframe. When spring arrives you won't need to think, or strain; the work will just flow. All you need to do is trust the menstrual force to deliver you to where you need to be.

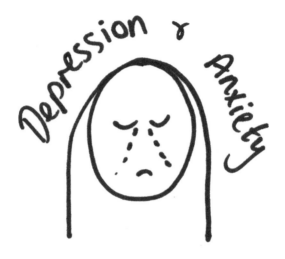

Depression & Anxiety

During the premenstrual and menstrual phases, depression and anxiety can worsen. If you feel suicidal during this time or your symptoms cause major disruption in your life on a regular basis, you may have premenstrual dysphoric disorder (PMDD). Seek help from your doctor.

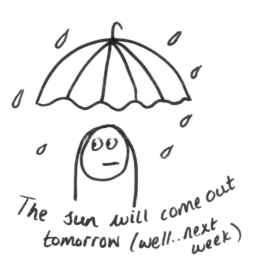

The sun will come out tomorrow (well...next week)

If you are struggling today and you are due on your period in a few days, stay strong. A coping strategy: make a list of the negative thoughts you are having; don't believe or disbelieve them, just write them down. Look at the list once your bleed is over. Is there anything you can do to address them? Any action you can take to make it easier next time PMS strikes?

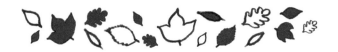

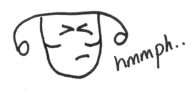

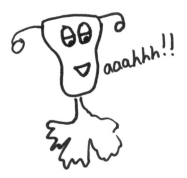

When you are overdue and waiting for your period to come, the tension in your body can be palpable, waiting for the sweet release. How can we harness that tension? Where can we find a productive use for that type of energy?

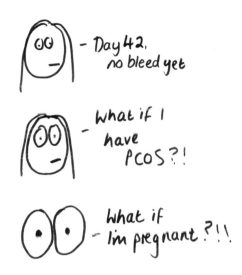

- Day 42, no bleed yet

- what if I have PCOS?!

- what if I'm pregnant?!!

Menstrual cycle length varies between women. Regular cycles that are 21 to 40 days long are normal (plus or minus 4 days' variation between average cycle length). Oligomenorrhea is the medical term for infrequent periods, and can be an indication of polycystic ovary syndrome (PCOS) but can also happen for many other reasons. It is common in the over 40s and under 15s. Or is it pregnancy?!

Diving
Deeper

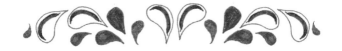

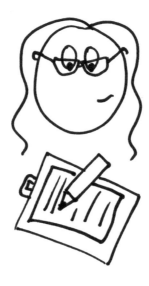

The inner seasonal archetypes are a great starting point for understanding the fluctuating energies of the menstrual cycle, but there is a great deal of variability between women and even between each cycle. The true challenge is to observe deeply what is happening in our own bodies without judgement.

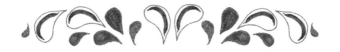

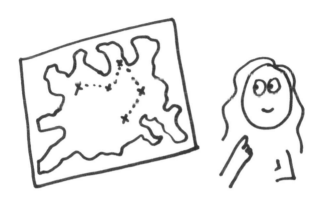

There are new paths to tread and new lessons to be learnt each cycle. What practise can we cultivate to stay in our bodies and out of our logical minds when practising menstrual cycle awareness? What journey will your cycle take you on this month?

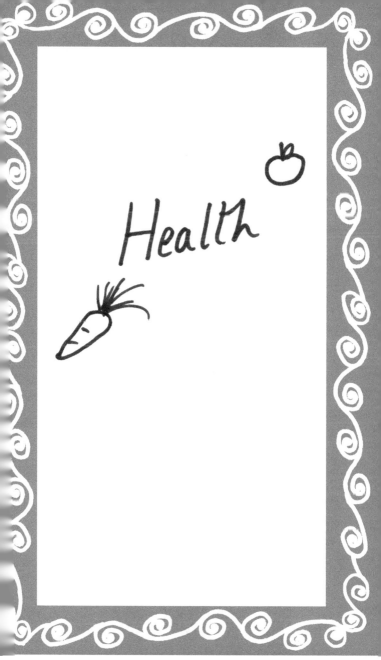

Health

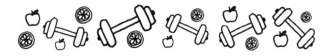

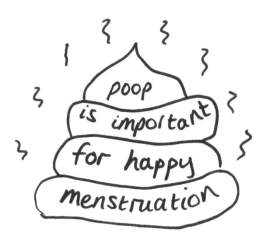

Gut health is important for good menstrual health. A healthy gut keeps food in the intestine and out of the blood stream (thus reducing inflammation in the body), promotes a healthy weight and metabolism, helps with the absorption of minerals and gets rid of toxins. Look after your friendly bacteria and poop well, friends!

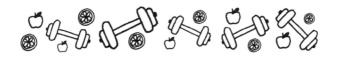

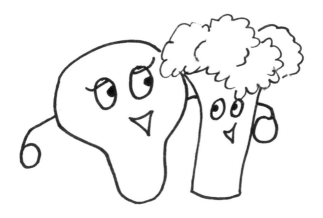

Cruciferous vegetables are a womb's best friend.
They are packed full of goodness, aid digestion and
contain nutrients that stimulate liver function,
helping to keep the menstrual cycle healthy.
Eating well is important to keep body fat levels
under control. High body fat is linked to insulin
resistance, which can cause cycle problems. Dietary
improvements are essential in addressing
menstrual problems.

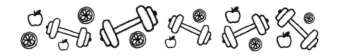

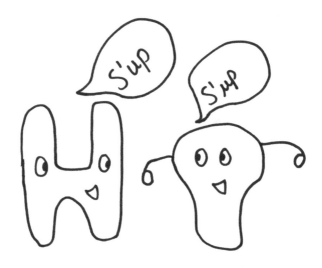

Your thyroid and your womb love to chat. The hormones that govern the menstrual cycle affect thyroid function and thyroid function can affect their production. It's part of the beautiful interweaving of systems that makes women so wondrous. Unfortunately, this may mean that a hormonal imbalance results in feelings of tiredness due to thyroid issues.

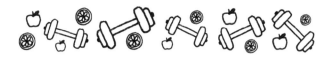

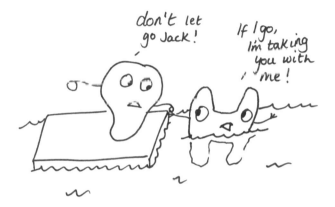

It also means that thyroid problems can mess with your cycle. Seek medical advice if you think there may be an issue with your thyroid.

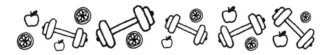

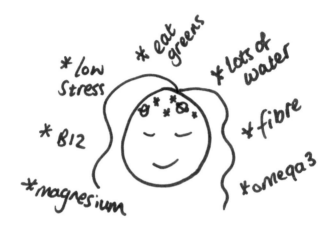

* low Stress
* eat greens
* lots of water
* B12
* fibre
* magnesium
* omega3

What vitamins and minerals do you need at which phase of the cycle? The real answer is you need all of them, all of the time. Eating for a healthy menstrual cycle is a month-long goal. There is some evidence that PMS is associated with low levels of B vitamins, magnesium, zinc, calcium and vitamin D. Eating a good, colourful diet all month round with lots of omega-3 is the best bet.

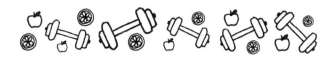

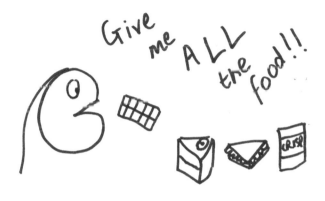

The premenstrual phase can bring about the serious munchies. However, balancing blood sugars is important for avoiding PMS, as insulin running riot after sugar binges can make you feel rubbish. Eating complex carbs and lots of protein as well as eating little and often may reduce cravings. Bla bla bla. Hand over the cookies!

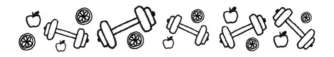

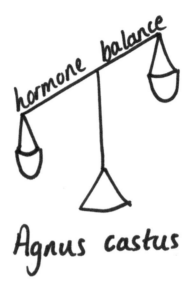

Agnus castus

There are many herbs that can help with menstrual cycle problems. Agnus castus is a good all-rounder for balancing hormone levels to reduce PMS symptoms.

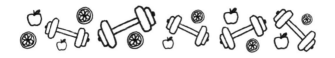

Milk Thistle

-helps liver function

Milk thistle is good for liver function, aiding good hormonal balance. Consulting a qualified herbalist is a good idea before you take anything.

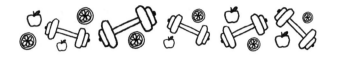

Period pain is one of the major reasons why people fall out with their wombs quite early on. The pain is caused by the womb being a bit too effective at contracting and chemical messengers called prostaglandins. Pain in early menstruating years doesn't usually have an underlying cause, but contact your doctor if it's so bad that it interferes with normal life. It should get better with age.

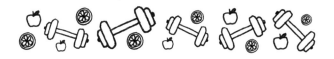

Once you have been having periods for a few years, if you experience menstrual pain, especially if it seems to be getting worse, there could be an underlying issue such as endometriosis, adenomyosis, fibroids, or something else. Trust your instinct, see a doctor and demand to be heard. Early detection is often important. After a certain age, periods should not be painful.

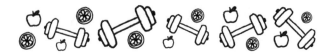

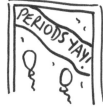

The prostaglandin Po-Po can really poop the period party with a pain-packing punch. NSAIDs (non-steroidal anti-inflammatory drugs) may help. Women have reported that rest, heat packs, massage, acupuncture and other remedies have helped them, but you need to find what works for you.

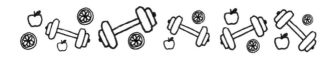

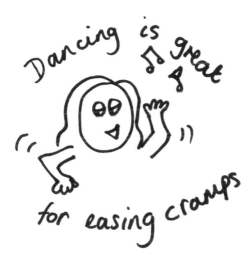

Dancing is my personal favourite activity for easing menstrual discomfort. Rolling, swaying moves leading from the pelvis are lovely. Sink right into your womb space. Eating chocolate cake at the same time really enhances the experience. Groove to the sound of those neurons firing. Celebrate the miracle of life and the sacredness of woman, from whom all human life flows.

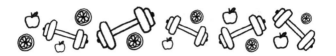

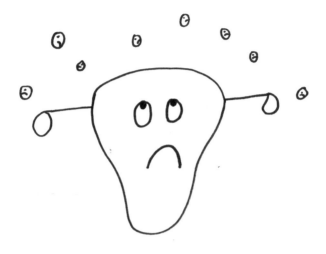

Endometriosis is a condition whereby cells like the ones in the lining of the womb are found elsewhere in the body. During menstruation they behave just like the cells of the womb lining, but the blood cannot escape.

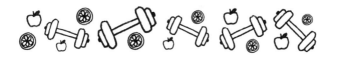

It is a very painful and debilitating condition and massively under-diagnosed. Fertility issues can arise.

Adenomyosis occurs when the lining of the womb is found in the muscle of the womb. It has similar symptoms to endometriosis.

If you regularly have heavy, painful periods, pain during sex, pelvic pain, painful bowel movements, fatigue, or pain days before your period, it is a good idea to see your doctor. Keep a journal of symptoms for information.

The earlier these problems are identified, the easier they are to deal with, so do not hesitate in contacting your doctor.

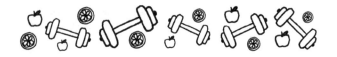

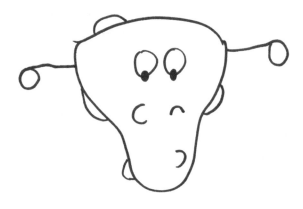

Fibroids are benign growths that develop in the uterus wall. They are very common and not usually a problem, but in some people they can cause issues such as heavy or painful bleeds, lower back pain, impact on bladder, constipation or pain during sex. Black women are disproportionately affected. Treatments are available so please see a doctor ASAP with concerns.

96

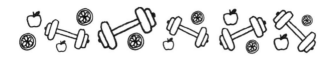

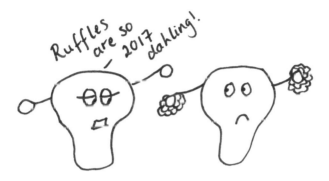

Polycystic ovary syndrome (PCOS) is a hormone disorder with an array of symptoms. Often, a large number of small cysts occur on the ovaries, due to eggs beginning to develop, but failing to be released. Symptoms can include irregular or no periods, heavy periods, excess body hair, hair loss on head, acne, pelvic pain, weight gain and fertility issues. A healthy diet can help, but the exact cause of PCOS is unknown and often runs in families. Consult your doctor for more information.

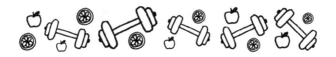

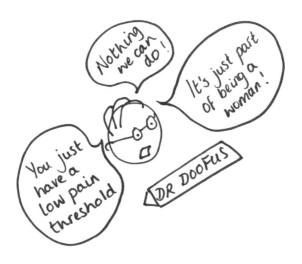

Unfortunately, there are still many doctors out there who do not take women's pain seriously. If you are not 100% happy with your doctor's response to your concerns, you are entitled to seek a second opinion.

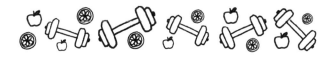

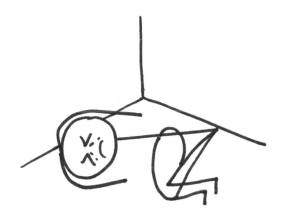

Period pain is the worst. I want you to know that it's not your fault. You have been let down from every angle; the taboo that stops you claiming the rest you need to help with the pain, the research that hasn't been done, sexual trauma, medical misogyny that continuously fuels the dismissal of our realities and the pervasive myth that periods are supposed to be painful.

Suggestions for minimising period pain:

- Rest as much as possible during your bleed.

- Eat more cruciferous vegetables (broccoli, cabbage etc.) throughout the month.

- Eat plenty of other fresh fruit and vegetables, fibre, omega-3 sources and drink lots of water. Cut down on alcohol, sugar, caffeine and unhealthy fatty foods.

- Boost healthy gut bacteria with fermented foods e.g. homemade sauerkraut.

- Try cutting out soy and dairy (or anything that causes inflammation of your gut).

- Minimise exposure to toxins and plastics.

- Find a type of exercise you enjoy doing.

- Reduce stress in your life where possible.

- Track your cycle; get to know your body.

- Seek therapy for sexual or birth trauma.

- Go for an abdominal massage.

- Use pads instead of tampons.

- Seek medical help if pain is excessive or if dietary changes are ineffective.

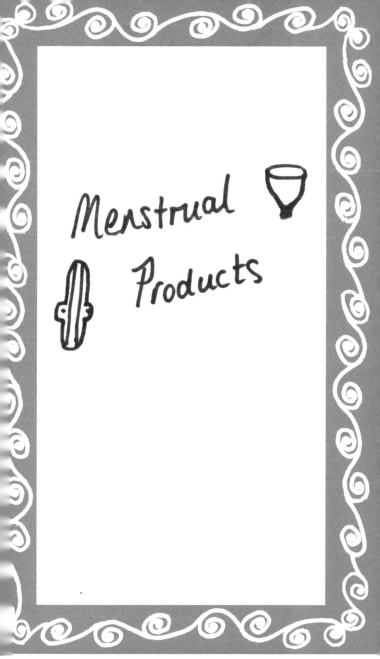

Menstrual Products

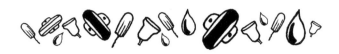

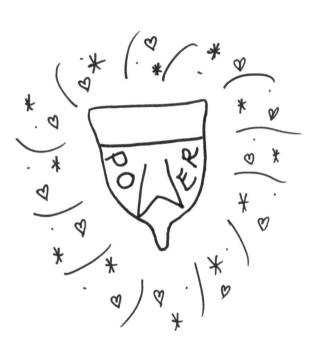

Holding a mooncup in your hand and seeing your blood is a major turning point for many women in how they feel about their periods. The power in your blood is palpable; its life-nourishing energy seems to vibrate in your hand. It's incredible! Something you once thought of as icky becomes amazing. I'll never forget the first time I experienced this.

Your blood can nourish and sustain new life. It's the part of you that midwives the soul to the physical world. It's a physical, touchable, real representation of just how powerful women are.

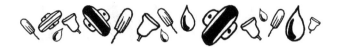

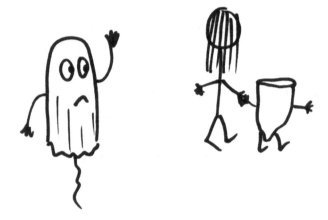

I never looked back.

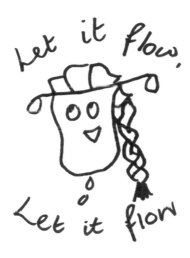

Let it flow,
Let it flow

Menstruation can be a really nice experience if you get the chance to just chill and let it flow.
Tampons can block your chi. They aren't great for the psyche or the vagina. Stick one in your mouth and you'll see why! Even mooncups can be party poopers. There's nothing quite like just letting it flow.

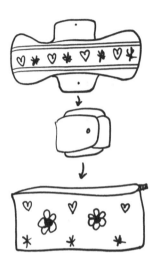

What to do with washable pads when you are out and about? They can be folded up, secured with their popper and stored in pretty waterproof bags. Cloth pads don't smell; they are lovely and soft on the vulva and won't expose it to any nasty plastics or chemicals. They are such a winner all round.

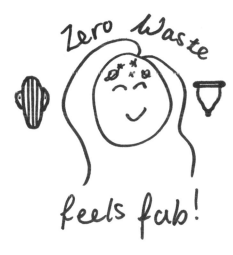

Zero Waste

feels fab!

It's such an amazing feeling to know that your menstrual products don't add anything to landfill. It's great on the pocket too! When the cloth pad matches the underwear, then it's really time to strut.

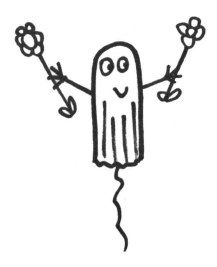

If reusable products are not for you, there are organic disposable products available which are very reasonably priced and free from pesticides or bleaches.

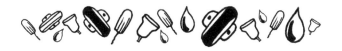

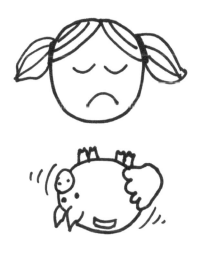

Even the cheapest menstrual products can become expensive. Period poverty is a massive problem globally that prevents girls from accessing education and holds them back. 10% of girls surveyed in the UK reported being unable to afford menstrual products. Thankfully, there are many charities and organisations working to change this.

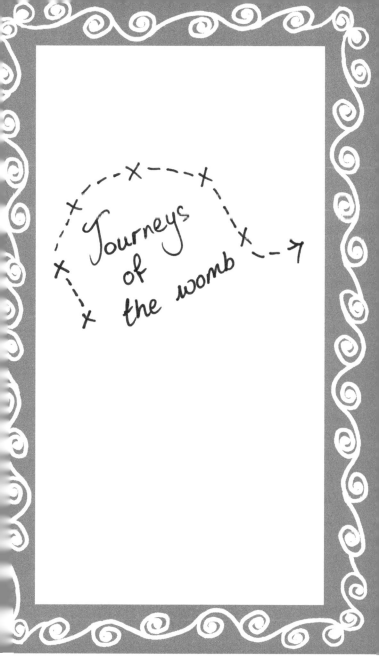

Journeys
of
the womb

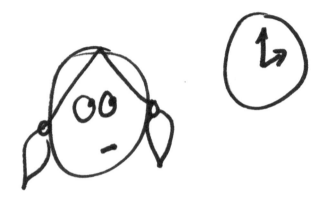

It can seem frustrating waiting for your first period, a strange mix of wanting it to come but also uncertainty about what to expect.

Remember, your body is beautiful; it does its own thing in its own time and nothing that comes out of your womb is ever disgusting, so don't let anyone make you feel that way.

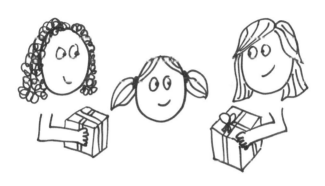

The first period, also called menarche, is a big moment in a girl's life. Marking this rite of passage with a ceremony can start the journey into womanhood off on the right note. Gifts can be exchanged, advice given and ritual performed to symbolise the crossing of this important threshold. Let's send our young women forward into their bleeding years full of joy and confidence.

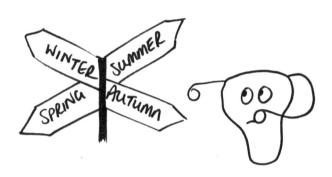

Your womb can take a while to settle into a cycle after your first period or birth/ breastfeeding. Eventually, when menopause approaches, cycles go astray. All these big transition moments can cause inner seasons to become unpredictable. If your cycle has gone haywire for no apparent reason, are you undergoing a big emotional transition moment in your life?

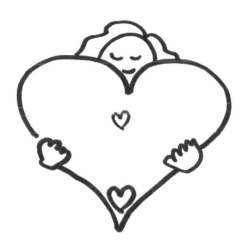

How much do you love your vulva? Vulvas come in all shapes and sizes. Around half of women have labia minora (inner labia) that are longer than the labia majora (outer labia) and perfect symmetry is very rare in nature. Check out some of the fantastic vulva galleries on the internet. Shame around female organs is so rife and unnecessary. All of you is beautiful.

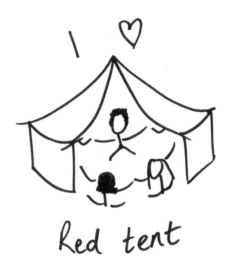

Red tent

The red tent movement is based on the ancient traditions of moon lodges, where women would go to menstruate together. We are now reviving the practise of coming together to release in a way that works for us in modern times. It's more about emotional release now, supporting women through all of life's journeys. Red tents are amazing. Time out with other women; time to just be.

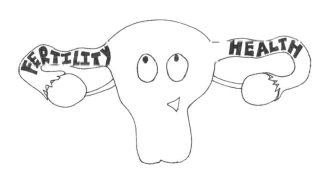

Fertility and womb health are linked and problems with periods can lead to fertility issues. I hope with better education we can nip menstrual problems in the bud, addressing issues early on so that fewer women have to experience the stress and heartbreak of fertility problems.

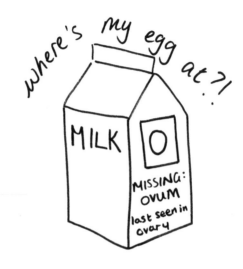

where's my egg at?!

MILK

MISSING:
OVUM
last seen in
ovary

Anovulatory cycles occur when no egg is released, characterised by very long or very short cycles. It is common in the first few menstruating years and when heading towards perimenopause. It can also happen if physical or emotional stress is affecting hormone levels, or for some other reason.

If you are trying for a baby menstrual cycle irregularities can be frustrating. Waiting for your womb to decide she wants another try, who knows how long she'll be on strike for?

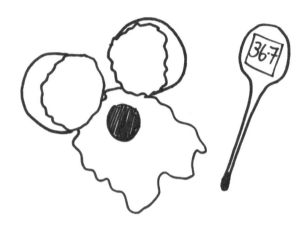

How do you know when you have ovulated? After ovulation your basal body temperature (BBT) increases by 0.2 to 0.5 degrees C. Cervical mucus becomes egg white-like when most fertile and changes in cervix position occur. Combine all these signs to get a clearer picture. Pee sticks are also available but aren't great for the environment.

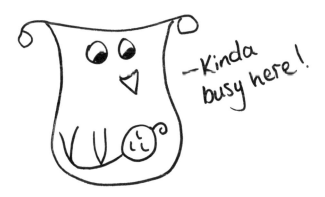

I'm always blown away by the power of the womb. The things she can do! She guides you through life by changing your inner seasons, ensuring you pay sufficient detail to every aspect of your existence. She truly shines during pregnancy, growing and loving a baby from an egg to a ready-to-face-the-world little human. We women have such incredible power within us; we are strength incarnate.

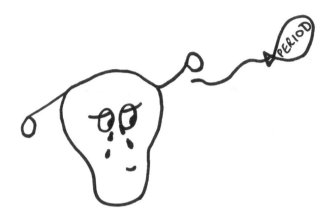

Perimenopause can be a bitter sweet time. On one hand there is the excitement of life beyond the trappings of reproductive biology, free from the inconvenience of periods and the demands sex drive can place on life, but on the other is the grief of saying goodbye to the ovulation highs, the sensual menstrual surrender and other personal magical moments from the cycle.

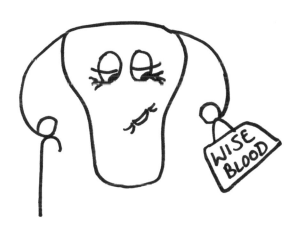

When you are wise enough to let go, when you are wise enough to find ways to release without your body setting monthly reminders, only then are you ready to hold onto your wise blood and pass through the gates of menopause. Your womb may be old, but you are not, and life has so much more to give.

Coming soon...

Goddess Doodles

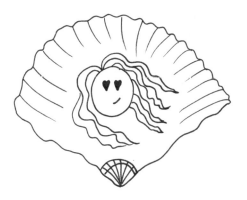

Support Organisations

Endometriosis UK
www.endometriosis-uk.org
0808 808 2227

Verity (PCOS support charity)
www.verity-pcos.org.uk

British Fibroid Trust
www.britishfibroidtrust.org.uk

National Association for Premenstrual Syndrome NAPS
www.pms.org.uk
0844 8157311

Mind (mental health charity)
www.mind.org.uk

Thyroid UK
thyroiduk.org.uk

British Thyroid Foundation
btf-thyroid.org

References

Cycle Length

Cole, L. A., *et al.* 2009. The normal variabilities of the menstrual cycle. *Fertility and Sterility.* 91: 522–527.

NHS (2010). Periods and fertility in the menstrual cycle. www.nhs.uk/conditions/periods/fertility-in-the menstrual-cycle/

Gut Health

Liu, R., *et al.* 2017. Dysbiosis of gut microbiota associated with clinical parameters in Polycystic Ovary Syndrome. *Front Microbiol.* 8: 324.

Guo, X., *et al.* 2017. High fat diet alters gut microbiota and the expression of paneth cell-antimicrobial peptides preceding changes of circulating inflammatory cytokines. *Mediators Inflamm.* Vol 2017 Article ID 9474896.

Cruciferous vegetables

Higdon, J.V., *et al.* 2007. Cruciferous vegetables and human cancer risk: epidemiologic evidence and mechanistic basis. *Pharmacol res.* 55: 224-236.

The Liver

Tsuchiya, Y., 2005. Cytochrome P450-mediated metabolism of estrogens and its regulation in human. *Cancer Lett.* 28;227(2):115-24

Thyroid Health

Stavreus Evers, A. 2012. Paracrine interactions of thyroid hormones and thyroid stimulation hormone in the female reproductive tract have an impact on female fertility. *Front Endocrinol (Lausanne).* 3: 50.

Singla, R., *et al.* 2015. Thyroid disorders and polycystic ovary syndrome: An emerging relationship. *Indian J Endocrinol Metab.* 19: 25– 29.

Shapiro, T.A., *et al.* 2006. Safety, tolerance, and metabolism of broccoli sprout glucosinolates and isothiocyanates: a clinical phase I study. *Nutr Cancer.* 55: 53-62.

Nutrients for PMS

Stewart, A., 1987. Clinical and biochemical effects of nutritional supplementation on the premenstrual syndrome. *J Reprod Med.* 32:435-41.

Bertone-Johnson, ER., *et al.* 2005. Calcium and vitamin D intake and risk of incident premenstrual syndrome. *Arch Intern Med.* 165(11):1246–1252.

Posaci, C., *et al.* 1994. Plasma copper, zinc and magnesium levels in patients with premenstrual tension syndrome. *Acta Obstetricia et Gynecologica Scandinavica.* 73: 452-455.

Herbs

Ceerqueira, R.O., *et al.* 2017. *Vitex agnus castus* for premenstrual syndrome and premenstrual dysphoric disorder: a systematic review. *Arch Womens Ment Health* 20(6):713-719

Hardy, M.L., 2000. Herbs of special interest to women. *J Am Pharm Assoc (Wash).* 40(2):234-42.

Insulin Resistance

Diamanti-Kandarakis, E., and Dunaif, A. (2012). Insulin resistance and the polycystic ovary syndrome revisited: an update on mechanisms and implications. *Endocrine Reviews.* 33(6), 981–1030.

A Note To My Generation

I believe the menstrual cycle is a magnificent gift, and problems arising with it should, for the large part, be solvable with the right support. Having said that, there comes a point where things have gone on for so long, and become so complicated, that hormonal medicine or a hysterectomy is the only way to get through the day. Unfortunately, this is the story for far too many women of my generation.

I hope our daughters will have a better chance at a healthy menstrual cycle. I hope we are able to guide them through relationship matters, nutritional changes to improve PMS and period pain and that our hard-earned emotional literacy can transfer to them so they can become boundaried, powerful and authentic people. I hope they receive far better medical care far earlier on.

Our generation has much work to do to turn things around, to give the gifts our mothers were unable to bestow upon us as their generation was busy fighting on other fronts. Their struggles have given us the ground upon which to hold this conversation today, and we must pass the baton to the next generation who will face new challenges, such as overcoming porn culture and ever-increasing environmental pollution.

All we can do is heal ourselves as much as possible, and lay the foundations for their future as best we can, by working together and re-centring the womb in the psyche of mankind.

Acknowledgements

I would like to thank my parents for being so wonderful and the rest of my family and family-in-law for always being there for me. A special thanks to my husband for his support and love.

Thank you to all my friends/test subjects who helped to perfect this work and my Facebook hive mind, who always came up with the solutions to various problems. Nicky Blecha's expert eye improved this book tenfold; my thanks go out to her.

My red tent sisters held and inspired me during the process and for them I am eternally grateful. Melonie Syrett (meloniesyrett.org), Rachael Crow (Moon Times), Leora Leboff and Kate Codrington (Woman Kind) prompted me to dive deeper with my cycle awareness practice and gave me the support and encouragement I needed to start this book. Thank you for walking beside me on this journey.

Thank you to all the wonderful authors from whom I learnt the gift of menstruality: Lara Owen, Miranda Gray, Melanie Swan, Alexandra Pope and Sjanie Hugo Wurlitzer of Red School.

An enormous thank you to all the women out there working on the menstrual cycle who aren't afraid to delve into the emotional aspects, who are fearsome in the face of the patriarchal oppression of women's bodies and bring heart into conversations dominated by heads.

About the Author

Becky became fascinated by the menstrual cycle during an uncomfortable pregnancy when she realised how much she missed it. She has always been interested in the human body, pursuing a career in cancer research until she left to become a full-time mother. She facilitates red tent women's circles, runs workshops on the menstrual cycle and leads menarche ceremonies. Becky lives in the UK with her husband and two children.

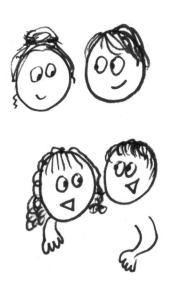